BACKPACKER.

Fitness & Nutrition for Hiking

Molly Absolon

T0352601

FALCON GUIDES

GUILFORD, CONNECTICUT
HELENA, MONTANA

In memory of AJ, Andy, and Rusty

FALCONGUIDES®

An imprint of Rowman & Littlefield

BACKPACKER is a registered trademark of Active Interest Media.
Falcon and FalconGuides are registered trademarks and Make Adventure Your
Story is a trademark of Rowman & Littlefield.

Distributed by NATIONAL BOOK NETWORK

British Library Cataloguing-in-Publication Information available

Library of Congress Cataloging-in-Publication Data is available on file.

ISBN 978-1-4930-1960-1 (paperback)
ISBN 978-1-4930-2372-1 (e-book)

∞™ The paper used in this publication meets the minimum requirements of
American National Standard for Information Sciences—Permanence of Paper for
Printed Library Materials, ANSI/NISO Z39.48-1992.

The author, *BACKPACKER* magazine, and Rowman & Littlefield
assume no liability for accidents happening to, or injuries sustained by,
readers who engage in the activities described in this book.

Contents

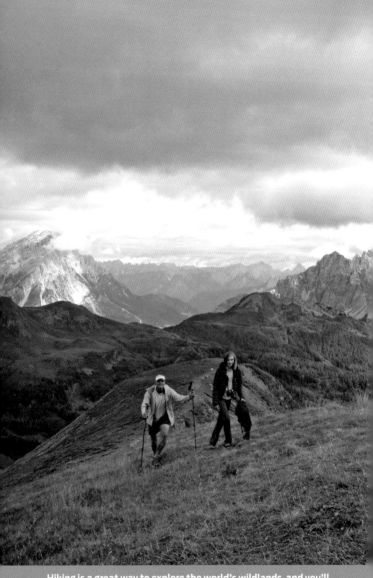

Hiking is a great way to explore the world's wildlands, and you'll enjoy it more if you are fit. MOLLY ABSOLON

Introduction

So you want to go backpacking. Maybe it's been a dream you've entertained for a long time. Maybe you saw the movie *Wild* or have been flipping through *BACKPACKER* recently and got inspired. Or maybe someone has invited you on a trip. Regardless of your motivation, backpacking through the wilderness is a great way to explore our nation's wildlands, and it doesn't demand extreme athleticism or years of training to enjoy.

Low skill and strength requirements do not mean that good fitness and nutrition aren't important, however. Most of us can get off the couch, don a pack, and walk a few miles down a trail, but chances are we won't have much fun after a while. As Nate Goldberg, the director of the Hiking Center at Beaver Creek Resort in Colorado, told Backpacker.com, "I've taken thousands of people into the mountains and the most elementary lesson I've learned is that there's an undeniable relationship between fitness and fun on the trail. The fitter you are, the more fun you have. End of story."

So if you want to enjoy your backcountry experience, it's a good idea to put a little energy into physical training before you head out. A mile can feel really long when your feet are sore and your body is tired. When you are fatigued, you end up trudging forward with your head down and your eyes focused on the

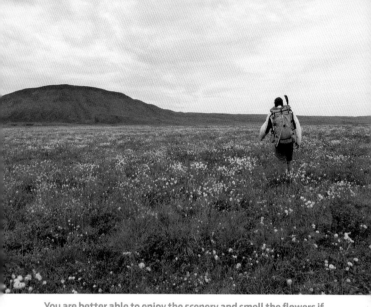

You are better able to enjoy the scenery and smell the flowers if you feel strong and comfortable when you hike. MOLLY ABSOLON

trail in front of you as you try to ease the weight of your backpack off your aching shoulders. In this condition it's easy to walk by a spectacular view or wildlife without even noticing. All you can think about is getting to the next rest stop or to camp, which kind of defeats the purpose of leaving home to begin with. If you are fit, you are better able to look around and enjoy your surroundings; plus, you'll have extra energy to climb a peak or go fishing when you reach your destination.

Strength, endurance, and good nutrition also help keep you safe and comfortable in the wilderness. You can move more easily around obstacles and maintain a good pace during a long day when you are fit. And good physical conditioning makes you feel more confident about your ability to achieve your goal and negotiate tricky terrain. It takes energy and strength to step down off a boulder or to clamber over a log across the trail. Training will help you perform these moves comfortably.

If you are weak and tired, on the other hand, you are more prone to discouragement, fear, and lack of

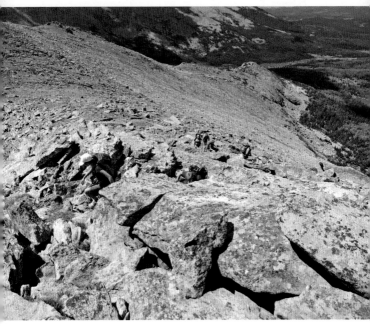

Good fitness allows you to negotiate tricky terrain with confidence. MOLLY ABSOLON

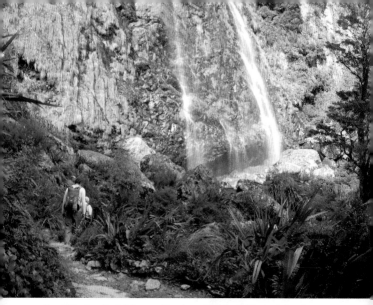

Conditioning for hiking and backpacking isn't like training for a marathon. You just want to be comfortable hiking through the mountains with a backpack on. MOLLY ABSOLON

confidence. You are also more likely to make mistakes or to fall, which could be dangerous. Finally, it's just no fun to hike in pain.

For these reasons, it's a good idea to do a little training before you head off on a hiking or backpacking trip. Don't let that idea intimidate you, however. We aren't talking about running a marathon at a competitive speed or going on a monthlong expedition to climb an 8,000-meter peak. We are talking about setting you up to walk through the mountains with a pack on and have a good time while doing it.

Chapter One

Before You Go

There are countless training regimens floating around these days. All of them promise extraordinary things: sleeker physiques, six-pack abs, bulging biceps, and the ability to leap tall buildings in a single bound. Some of the promises are hype, particularly if they claim you can achieve these outcomes with minimal effort. Some of them really will change how you look, feel, and perform.

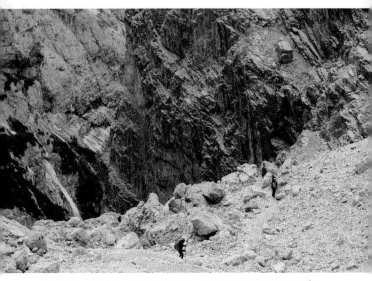

Taking a spin class or doing yoga is not going to prepare you for the ups and downs of hiking. To really get ready to hike, you need to hike. SCOTT KANE

The main thing to keep in mind when you are trying to pick a training program is your goal. If you want to go backpacking, taking a spin class at your local gym is probably not the best choice. You'll get strong on your bicycle, but that strength doesn't necessarily translate well to walking. You need a program that targets the muscles you'll use in your chosen activity, and you need to use those muscles in the way you intend to use them. So if you are going to go hiking, the very best way to train is to go hiking or to find activities that mimic hiking, such as stair climbing or step-ups. The main muscles you want to train are in your legs and butt: your quads, glutes, calves, and hamstrings. But your core plays an important role in stability as well, so don't neglect your abs and back as you prepare your body.

PERSONAL TRAINER VERSUS CLASSES VERSUS GOING ON YOUR OWN

This book will outline a basic training plan geared toward backpackers and hikers, but that may not be enough to get you motivated. Some people have no trouble setting a goal and sticking to it, even if they have to train alone at odd hours of the day. Others need to be in a class or to have a trainer or partner to egg them on.

Be realistic about yourself. If you have never kept a New Year's resolution in your life, there's a good chance you aren't going to stick to a training program on your own. If that sounds like you, you might benefit from the discipline and direction of a fitness class or a personal trainer. Look for basic strength building, core, and cardio options. You can tailor the specifics with some at-home work to ensure you are exercising the proper muscle groups. If you have a trainer, talk about your goals so he or she can design your program to help you achieve success.

If you don't have access to a gym or don't want to spend the money but are worried about staying committed to your goal, try to find a training partner. It's hard to skip a workout when you know somebody is waiting for you.

TIMELINE

The best way to figure out when to start training is to define your objective and then work backward. Let's say you want to take a weeklong trip averaging 6 to 10 miles per day. Most people hike about 2 mph with a loaded backpack on a trail. You may move faster over level terrain, but when you factor in rest breaks, elevation gain, and unexpected obstacles, 2 mph is a good starting point. So figure you will be on the trail for up to 5 hours or more a day. That means your training program should be geared toward that goal.

Assuming you are basically starting from zero, you will want to build gradually to that level of activity.

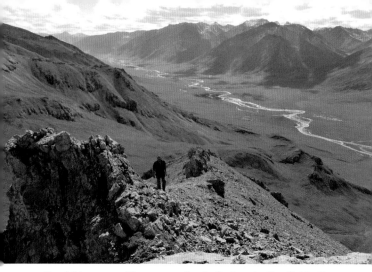

Your hiking pace will vary according to the terrain. On a flat trail you can hike 2 to 3 miles per hour with a pack on. Hiking off-trail or ascending steep terrain will slow you down. MOLLY ABSOLON

For the goal outlined above, six to eight weeks should give you plenty of time.

COMPONENTS OF A GOOD TRAINING PROGRAM

A well-rounded training program geared toward backpacking and hiking will include endurance or cardio training, strength building, interval workouts, mobility or core exercises, and rest.

» Endurance or cardio activities build up your stamina and toughen up your body for the wear and tear of a long day. The philosophy of training is constantly evolving and today's conventional wisdom may not be tomorrow's, but in general most trainers say you do not have to grind out hours and hours of cardio training to achieve a good level of fitness. But it is important to build up to the point where you do at least one workout that lasts as long as you anticipate you'll be exercising on your hiking excursion—this ensures you have the physical and mental toughness to keep going even when you want to stop during your trip. For backpacking you want to know that you can hike comfortably with a pack on for 5 hours or more. The best way to find that out is to try it beforehand.

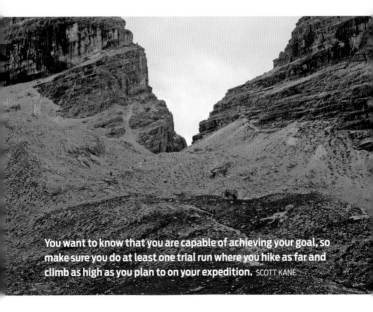

You want to know that you are capable of achieving your goal, so make sure you do at least one trial run where you hike as far and climb as high as you plan to on your expedition. SCOTT KANE

» Strength building helps you develop stability and power. You don't need to do a lot of weight lifting to enjoy backpacking, but squats, step-ups, lunges, hamstring curls, and other strength-building activities help develop your leg muscles and core so that you can clamber over boulders or step off a stream bank with confidence. Keep body symmetry in mind as you develop your exercise routine. Our bodies work best when balanced—so don't just focus on your quads. You need to work the opposing muscle group—in this case your hamstrings—as well to ensure they complement each other properly. Imbalance can lead to long-term problems like osteoarthritis, tendonitis, and back pain, or short-term athletic injuries like sprains or strains.

A 2008 study by researchers at the Norwegian University of Science and Technology compared distance runners who performed squats in the gym three times a week with others who followed their normal running regimen without any strength training. The findings were startling. The gym goers improved their running economy and extended the time it took for them to become exhausted at maximal aerobic speed by 21 percent. The runners who did not hit the gym saw no change in their performance. These findings

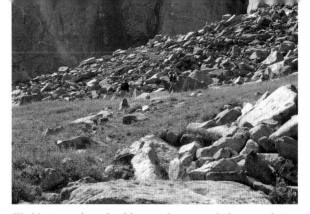

Climbing up and over boulders requires power, balance, and stability, all of which can be developed through strength training at the gym a few days a week. KATHY BROWN

reinforce the fact that performing strength-building exercises a few times a week will improve your performance in the field. Start with light loads and build gradually. Consult a professional to ensure the exercises you perform are targeted toward your final goal.

» Mobility and core exercises ensure that your muscles are supple and your body is balanced. All movement originates in the core, so a strong core is integral to everything from proper posture to good walking technique. Adding a few minutes of core exercises and stretches to the end of your workout helps improve balance and tone, increases your mobility, and makes you less prone to injury.

» Rest is also key to a good training program. If you jump into a new fitness regimen too vigorously, chances are you will get stiff and sore, making it hard to continue to exercise. A little soreness is not bad, but if it affects your ability to maintain your training, you need to cut back. Overtraining can also lead to mental and physical fatigue: You just don't feel like working out anymore. To avoid overdoing it, build a rest day into your program to give your body time to recuperate.

ADDING WEIGHT

The one thing that will set a backpacking/hiking training program apart from other regimens is the addition of weight. To really prepare for a hiking trip, you have to get used to carrying a backpack, and that takes some practice.

Your backpack doesn't have to be extremely heavy. Today's outdoor gear is light. There are backpackers who routinely carry packs that weigh less than 20 pounds on multiday trips. Minimizing your pack weight is a great goal, but even 20 pounds on your back can get tiring if you aren't used to carrying it.

To prepare for the additional weight, start carrying your backpack when you are performing your cardio or endurance workouts. You can start light—say 10 pounds—and add weight until you are carrying 20 to 30 pounds. One trick is to fill your pack

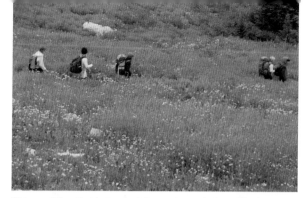

The one thing that sets a training regimen designed for back-packing apart from a general fitness program is the need to get used to carrying a pack. Carry some weight in your backpack when you do your training hikes to build tolerance and strength.
MOLLY ABSOLON

with a couple of full water bottles or water bladders to weigh it down. That way, on your descent, you can dump out the water to save your knees. (A quart of water weighs about 2.2 pounds.)

KEEP A TRAINING LOG

If you really want to ensure that your training regimen gets you ready for your backpacking trip, keep a train-ing log. It's easy to go out and jog around the block a few times, but if you don't up the ante over time, your training will quickly plateau and all you'll really have prepped to do is run around that block. To gain strength and endurance, you need to keep increasing your workload by adding speed, weight, or distance to your program.

Track your daily workouts, making notes on times, distances, and weight. Try to build on these milestones. If it takes you an hour and a half to walk up a nearby mountain one week, see if you can cut a few minutes off that time the next week, or throw some 30-second, maximum-intensity intervals into the mix. You don't even have to use a watch: just speed up your walking or break into a sprint and count out 30 seconds. (You know how to do that: 1-Mississippi, 2-Mississippi, and so forth.) When you hit 30, slow your pace and get your heart rate down for approximately 1 minute, then do another 30-second sprint. Start with three intervals and add more as you get stronger. Or try to maintain your sprint for longer. Either way it adds value to your hike without taking extra time.

It's easy to fall into a training rut, especially when you have time constraints. Tracking your progress and adding challenges helps keep you motivated and out of a rut.

Sample Training Regimen

Monday	Tuesday	Wednesday	Thursday	Friday	Saturday	Sunday
Rest and recovery	Strength /gym	Cardio	Strength /gym	Cardio	Long endurance hike	Cross-training

YOUR WORKOUT

The length of time you spend on your training really depends on your schedule and base fitness level.

If you are just starting out, shoot for 30 minutes of exercise per session for your first week, except on Saturday, when you should head out for a 45-minute walk. Add to your time as you gain fitness until you are working out for 1 hour and hiking all day. (If you have never exercised before, are obese, or have health concerns, you should consult a physician before you begin a training program. This book is geared toward people who are active but want to do some specific training to improve their performance backpacking.)

In general you can add 15 to 20 percent to your workout times each week. So if you are starting at 30 minutes, add 5 minutes or so every week to your workout time. If you find that this increase is too much, slow down. If it's too easy, bump it up a little. Your goal is to push yourself and work hard. It's fine to get a little stiff occasionally, but getting really sore is often counterproductive because it keeps you from training hard the next go-round, so build up the intensity and duration of your workouts gradually.

If your schedule does not allow you to hit the gym for an hour every day, 15 to 20 minutes of intense exercise is still beneficial, so don't skip your workout just because you are short on time.

Gym Workouts (Tuesday and Thursday)

Hiking trails are rarely flat and smooth once you leave your city park. If you plan to head into the mountains, you'll be scrambling around boulders, hiking up and down steep sections of trail, clambering over logs, and crossing streams. These movements demand balance, power, and strength, all of which can be developed in the gym.

Start with a 5-minute warm-up. This can include walking or jogging on a treadmill or stair climber or rowing at a moderate pace on a rowing machine. You just want to get your heart rate up a little bit.

Mobility Exercises

Next, go through the following series of mobility exercises to get your joints moving and your blood flowing. It's a good idea to go through this series before you start hiking, too. These exercises should take about 10 minutes.

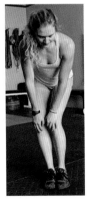

Warm up your joints with gentle rotations.

AVERY ABSOLON

1. Joint rotation: Stand tall and gently turn each ankle in a circle 8 times. Reverse. Next, place your hands on your thighs and swivel your knees around 8 times. Reverse. Place your hands on your hips and rotate your hips in a circle 8 times. Reverse. Circle your wrists 8 times in each direction. Gently turn your head to the left, then lower your chin to your chest, then look right. Reverse. Repeat 8 times in each direction.

2. Arm swings: With straight arms, swing your arms back and forth in a scissoring motion. Do this 8 times for each arm.

3. Arm circles: Gently make small forward circles with your arms 8 times. Reverse. Then do 8 large forward circles. Reverse.

4. Back-to-wall arm slides: Stand with your heels and back against the wall. Place your arms out to your sides at shoulder height, elbows bent to 90 degrees and pressed against the wall. Slide your hands up

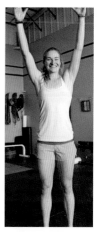

Circle your arms to help loosen up your shoulders.
AVERY ABSOLON

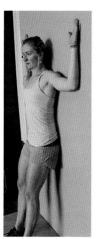
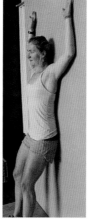

Stand against the wall with your back flat, elbows bent at 90 degrees. Slide your arms up and over your head, keeping your back pressed against the wall. Lower and repeat. This exercise helps improve shoulder mobility.
AVERY ABSOLON

the wall, straightening your arms until they are extended overhead. Try to keep your hands, arms, shoulders, and back flat against the wall. Lower and repeat 8 times.

5.   Upper back rotation: Get onto your hands and knees. Place one hand behind your head, rotate that elbow down and under your body to meet the other elbow, then twist back so that elbow is facing the ceiling. Do 8 repetitions, and then switch sides and do 8 repetitions on the other side. Your eyes should follow your elbow. Your hips and legs should remain motionless. Finish with 8 cat-cow movements, where you move between an arched back and a sway back in time with your breath.

6.   Side-to-side lunge: Start with your feet twice shoulder-width apart, feet facing straight ahead. Clasp your hands in front of your chest. Step out to the side with your right leg, shifting your entire weight onto that foot and sinking down so that your right knee is bent at a 90-degree angle (or less). Push your hips backward and keep your back flat. Your left leg will be straight. Return to your starting position and repeat on the opposite side. Do 8 repetitions per side.

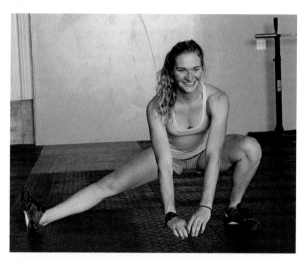

To do a side-to-side lunge, step out to one side and sink down into a squat with your opposite leg extended. Return to center and repeat on the opposite side. Side-to-side lunges help develop lateral strength and require the use of small stabilizing muscles that are essential to balance on the trail. AVERY ABSOLON

7. Inchworm: Bend over and place your hands on the floor in front of you. Walk your hands out until you are in a plank position, where your body is parallel to the ground balanced on your hands and toes, arms straight and in line with your shoulders. Take tiny steps in with your feet, keeping your knees straight until you return to your starting position. Repeat 8 times.

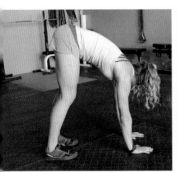
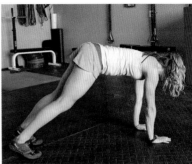
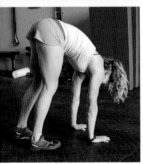
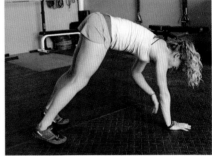

Start the inchworm in a standing position. Bend over until your hands are on the floor and then walk them out in front until you are in a plank position: body straight, parallel to the floor, hands beneath shoulders, arms straight, balanced on your hands and toes. Then walk your feet to your hands, stand up, and repeat. Inchworm wakes up all the muscles in your arms, shoulders, core, back, and legs. AVERY ABSOLON

Strength-building Exercises

Continue with more rigorous strength-building exercises to increase power and strength.

If you get bored with these exercises or they become too easy, you can look online for other options. Backpacker.com has training tips specifically designed for hikers. The following exercises are from backpacker.com.

1. Clockwork lunge: From a standing position, step forward with one leg, lowering your hips until both knees are bent at a 90-degree angle. Make sure the knee on your forward leg is straight above your toes. Step back to standing. Your starting point marks 12 o'clock. Now turn to 1 o'clock and, using the same leg, repeat your lunge. Continue around the clock until you return to 12. Now repeat the process, rotating counterclockwise and stepping forward with your opposite leg for each lunge. Lunges help strengthen your quadriceps and your glutes. Working in a circle helps you develop your ability to handle lateral steps and diagonal movements.

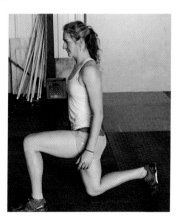

Make sure you maintain good form in your forward lunge. Your knees should be bent at a 90-degree angle. The forward knee should be in line with your toes and should extend straight out from your hip. Watch for inward rotation and overflexing at the ankle. AVERY ABSOLON

Up the ante by moving as quickly as you can through the lunges without losing your form. You can spring back to standing by pushing off on your forward leg. To make it even harder, put your backpack on and perform the lunges with weight on your back. Start with 10 pounds and build up. Remember, only add difficulty if you can maintain proper form.

2. One-leg calf raises: Your calves are integral to climbing steep hills efficiently, so it's important to pump them up for the challenge. Put a 45-pound weight plate on the floor or use a 2-inch-thick wooden board. Place your toes on the plate or plank and lower your heels to the ground. Curl one foot around the other ankle so you are balancing on one leg. Lift up onto your toes and lower. Do four sets of 25 repetitions for each leg, for a total of 100 calf raises per leg. Doing one-leg calf raises adds a balance component to the exercise and helps you develop stability.

Up the ante by following this exercise with a series of one-legged hops across an imaginary line on the ground. Do 100 per leg. Hopping strengthens your connective tissues and can help prevent sprains. But if you have joint issues, don't hop. Impact can be hard on joints, especially if you aren't strong enough to absorb some of the force with your muscles.

3. Hanging hip flexors: Hang from a chin-up bar with your arms and legs straight down. Bend your knees and lift them toward your chest while rotating to one side. Lower. Lift your knees again, this time twisting in the opposite direction. Do two sets of 10 on each side. This exercise helps strengthen your hip flexors, lower abdomen, and the oblique muscles in your core, all of which are important stabilizers when hiking.

Up the ante by adding a pull-up in between hip raises or increasing the number of repetitions per side to 15.

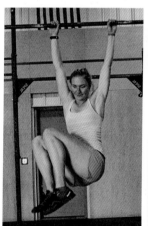
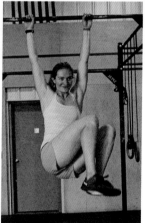

Hang from a chin-up bar with your arms and legs straight. Raise your knees to your chest while rotating to one side; lower and repeat on the opposite side. This is a great core exercise that helps keep you stable when negotiating obstacles on the trail.
AVERY ABSOLON

4. Bicycle crunches: Lie on your back, hands behind your head, elbows wide. Lift your shoulders off the floor, keeping your chin tucked down to your chest. Twist your torso, bringing your left elbow to your right knee and extending your left leg. Then repeat on the opposite side. Keep your feet flexed throughout. Do two sets of 30 (15 per side). These exercises help stabilize your core, which is where all your lower-body movements originate. The stronger your core, the better able you are to tackle challenging terrain and negotiate tricky obstacles.

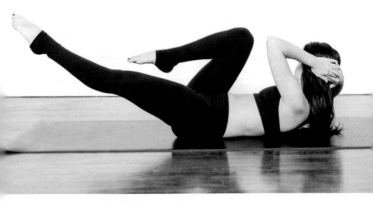

Bicycle crunches help strengthen your core. THINKSTOCK

5. Jumping jacks: Start by standing with feet together, arms at your sides. With a little hop spread your feet about shoulder width. At the same time raise your arms to the sides up above your head. With another hop, return your feet and arms to the starting position. That's one repetition. Do two sets of 25. Don't allow your knees to turn inward as you spread your feet apart—that will help you work your glutes to greatest advantage. Jumping jacks help you develop your coordination, agility, and explosive strength. The more coordinated you are, the smoother your jacks will be.

   Up the ante by jumping higher and faster and working up to 100 repetitions. If that is still too easy, drop to a lunge after you bring your feet together.

6. Burpees: The dreaded burpee is actually an excellent way to crank up the intensity of your training program. Burpees can be dialed down or up depending on how hard you want to go. For the basic burpee, start standing, then drop into a squat position, lower your hands to the ground, kick your legs out into a plank behind you, and drop down to the floor. Push back up into a plank, pull your feet back to your hands, and spring up, jumping off the ground with your hands overhead. Repeat. Do 25 burpees, rest for

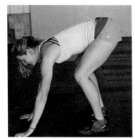
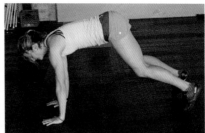
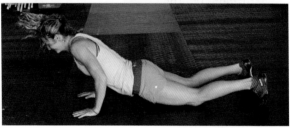
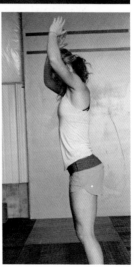

Burpees are a great all-body exercise that uses your core, your legs, and your shoulders. They also get your heart going. Start standing. Bend over and place your hands on the ground, jump your feet behind you into a plank, lower to the ground, and then reverse the sequence. AVERY ABSOLON

30 seconds, and repeat three times. If that's too much, you can do a simple squat thrust, where you jump your legs back into a plank but don't lower to the ground or jump up at the end. If you want more intensity, add a push-up when you are extended in a plank.

7. Hamstring curls: There are many ways to do a hamstring curl. The simplest is to lie flat on the ground, facedown, with a dumbbell in between your feet. (Start with 5 or 10 pounds and add weight as needed.) Bend your knees to 90 degrees, raising the weight between your feet. Lower and repeat. You can do two sets of 15 to 20 of these curls.

You can also do hamstring curls on a fitness ball. For this method, place your feet on top of the ball and raise your hips until you are in a reverse plank, shoulders on the ground. Bend your knees, pulling the ball in to your butt. Reverse. That's one repetition. Do 15 reps, rest, and repeat. Remember not to lower your hips throughout this exercise. You can add repetitions as you gain strength, but always make sure you move correctly throughout the sequence. Your hips should be even and high, and your back should be straight.

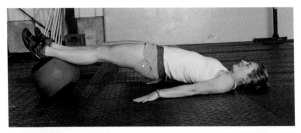

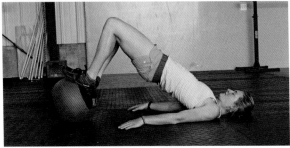

Hiking can be very quad intensive, so it's important to do exercises that target your hamstrings to ensure balance. There are many different ways to do hamstring curls. To do them with a fitness ball, lie down on your back with your feet on the ball. Raise your hips up off the ground. Make sure they are level. Roll the ball in to your butt and back out again. AVERY ABSOLON

Up the ante by doing deadlifts. You'll need a barbell for these exercises, but many trainers consider them to be the best way to target your hamstrings. Start with a light weight and build up the weight gradually to ensure you don't hurt yourself.

To do a deadlift, stand with your feet hip-width apart, knees slightly bent. Bend over with a flat back, pushing your hips back, and put your hands on the bar. Tighten your muscles, squeeze your butt, and stand, opening up at your hips and straightening your back and then your knees. To return the weight to the floor, push your hips back, fold at the hips, and then bend your knees. Repeat. Good form is critical. If you round your back, you can hurt it, so look in a mirror or have someone videotape you to ensure you are performing the exercise correctly. If you cannot maintain good form, switch to a lighter weight.

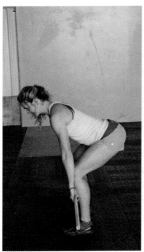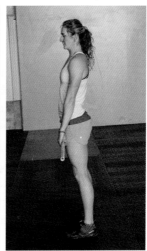

Deadlifts are a great way to strengthen your hamstrings, but they need to be done with proper form to ensure you do not get injured. Make sure your back stays flat. Start with the weight on the ground; from a standing position, bend over at the hips, keeping your back flat. Grab the bar, tighten your muscles, and stand, opening your back and hips and then straightening your knees. AVERY ABSOLON

8. Air squats: The ultimate exercise for developing your quads and glutes, air squats can be done anywhere at any time. There's a lot going on in a properly performed squat that provides additional benefits to your training beyond its obvious impact on your quads and glutes. Squats help increase the flexibility of your ankle joint and require good hip mobility. The muscles along your lumbar spine help maintain stability and prevent your lower back from rounding during a squat. Your upper back is also engaged to help maintain good posture. All together, these muscles work to help maintain balance, stability, and strength throughout your body.

    Stand with your feet hip-width apart, toes turned slightly outward. Push your butt and hips back and down, and bend your knees, lowering until your thighs are parallel to the floor with your arms extended straight in front of you. Make sure your knees remain over your toes, and do not collapse inward. Keep your torso upright and look ahead. Some people can go lower than 90 degrees, but make sure your body position remains good if you try. To stand up, squeeze your butt, straighten your legs, and lower your arms to your sides. Repeat. Start with three sets of 15 and increase as you gain strength and comfort.

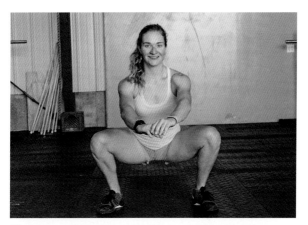

Air squats are a great way to build your glutes and quads, muscles that are essential to hiking and backpacking. Start in a standing position, knees hip-width apart, and lower your butt down until your knees are bent to 90 degrees or less. (The depth of your squat is determined by ankle flexibility.) Push your hips back and keep your back flat, eyes forward. Make sure your knees are above your toes and that they extend straight out from your hips. AVERY ABSOLON

Up the ante by wearing your backpack with 20 pounds or more inside. Or try a leg blaster routine where you do 25 air squats, 25 split squats (step forward into a lunge with both legs at 90 degrees, then repeat on the opposite side for one repetition), 25 jumping squats, and 25 jumping split squats. Only do this routine if you can maintain form and land lightly on the jumps. This involves a strong core. If you find yourself crashing down, don't jump.

Another way to make your squats more challenging is to do a goblet squat. You'll need a dumbbell or kettlebell for this exercise. Start with 15 pounds and build as you gain strength and stability. As always, only increase your weight if you can maintain good form throughout. To do a goblet squat, hold the weight against your chest, elbows out. Stand with your feet a bit wider than you would for a normal squat—just wider than shoulder-width apart. Then proceed with your normal squatting routine.

9. Bench hops: You'll need a bench-press bench for this exercise. Place a bar on the highest barbell setting on the rack. Stand to one side of the bench, and grab the bar so your hands are shoulder-width apart in the center of it. Squat down and jump up onto the bench, using your hands for stability. Keep your head up and eyes ahead, and make sure to engage your core as you jump. Try to make the landing light by squeezing your butt muscles and tightening your abs. Pause and then jump down on the opposite side of the bench. Reverse the sequence. That is 1 repetition. Do four sets of 6 with 1 to 2 minutes of rest in between.

    This explosive exercise requires maximal exertion and is a great way to develop power and strength. It's also a good metabolic workout and will get your heart rate up fast!

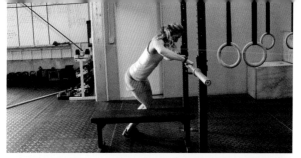
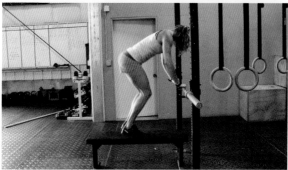
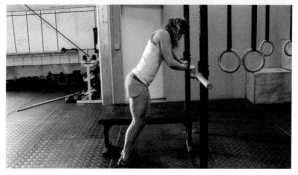

To perform a bench hop, use a bar for stabilization. Holding onto the bar, jump up and onto the bench, then down and off the other side. Repeat in the opposite direction. This exercise moves you laterally, recruiting some of the hard-to-get-to stabilizing muscles that are so critical to feeling balanced and strong on the trail. AVERY ABSOLON

Up the ante by doing box jumps without the barbell for support. Jump lightly onto a sturdy box that's anywhere from 15 to 24 inches in height. (Taller people may go even higher.) Make sure that you land on both feet squarely on top of the box, knees bent. Pause and step down off the box. The key is to make your landings light; you do that by engaging your core aggressively. Think: Squeeze your butt, tighten your abs. Start with 8 to 10 repetitions and build from there. Only add reps if you are maintaining good body position and control throughout. Do two to three sets with 1 to 2 minutes of rest in between.

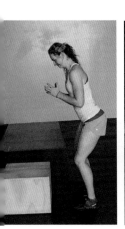 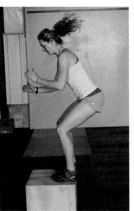 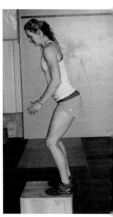

Box jumps are another explosive exercise that requires maximal exertion and rapid firing of your muscles to complete the move properly. Make sure that you land with both feet squarely on the box. Step down between jumps to avoid injury. Rest in between sets so that you are able to maintain proper form for each jump.

AVERY ABSOLON

If you don't want to jump, do step-ups with your backpack on. You can use a bench or box. Start with a height of 15 inches. Step up on top of the box, fully straightening your leg at the top. Bring your other leg up beside your first leg. Pause. Step down with the same leg. Repeat on the opposite side. Do 25 repetitions on each leg. Add weight or height to increase difficulty, but only if and when you can do the exercise with proper form and control.

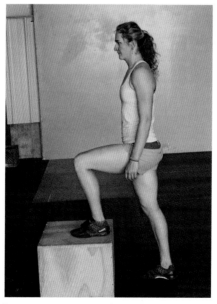

Not all of us are meant to jump. If you have joint issues or are just starting your fitness regimen, step-ups are more appropriate. Make sure that you step squarely on top of the box and pause before you step down. AVERY ABSOLON

10. Kettlebell swings: Kettlebell swings are an explosive exercise that engages your hips, lower back, glutes, hamstrings, and abdominal muscles, so you get a lot of bang for your buck from them. A properly performed swing comes from a hip snap and works best if you have consciously tightened up your core muscles. You will need a kettlebell or dumbbell to do this exercise. Start with 15 or 20 pounds (more for bigger, stronger individuals). Lighter weights help you avoid overloading your lower back. If the weight is too heavy, you may resort to using your back more than your hips, and that can lead to injury. So start light and build. You can always do more reps.

Stand with your feet hip-width apart, chest up, shoulders back and down, and the kettlebell hanging down, gripped loosely in your hands with your palms facing your body, arms straight. Engage your core, squeeze your butt, and retract your shoulder blades. Now you are ready. Drive through your heel, thrust your hips forward, and swing the weight up to chest height, arms extended. Let gravity help you lower the weight back to your starting position. Shift your weight back onto your heels, bend at the hips, and allow the kettlebell to swing down between your legs. Then explode forward again. Make sure that you are maintaining control throughout this exercise. To start out, do three sets of 15 repetitions. As you get comfortable with the exercise, you can use a heavier weight or increase the number of reps.

Up the ante by combining your kettlebell swings with a squat thrust, where you place your hands on the ground, kick back your legs into a plank, pull them back in, and return to standing. Do 15 swings, 15 squat thrusts, then 14 swings, 14 squat thrusts. Continue decreasing until you do 1 of each. Then you are done.

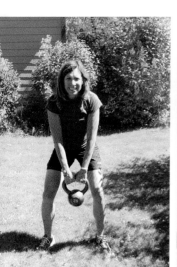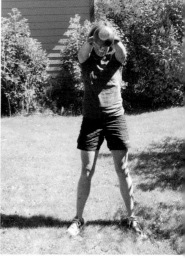

Kettlebell swings target a bunch of muscle groups that are key to strength, balance, and power. The key is to perform the swing properly. Always maintain a flat back and keep your arms straight, knees slightly bent, and eyes looking forward. Focus on getting the power for your swing from snapping your hips forward. AVERY ABSOLON

How to Design Your Workout

When you first start your training regimen, mix and match the exercises above. Think about complementary muscle groups as you pick your routine for the day. If you are doing a lot of squats and lunges, make sure to include hamstring curls. If you are working your abdomen hard, add some exercises that tone your back. Try to move through your routine quickly, with minimal rest in between exercises. Design a circuit that includes four or five exercises and repeat it three times, with 1-minute rest periods in between each circuit. As your fitness level improves, add exercises, increase the number of times through the circuit, or add weight to the exercises.

Cardio (Wednesday and Friday)

For your cardio training, go for a run or a brisk walk. Start at a moderate pace that allows you to carry on a conversation. If you haven't run or walked before, start with 30 minutes and add 20 percent every time you head out until you build to 1 hour. If you have some base level of fitness, you can start with 40 minutes.

Include a steep hill on your route that takes roughly 30 seconds to ascend. Ten minutes into your run/walk, sprint up that hill and then turn around and walk down. If you are out for just 30 minutes, do this twice. As your run/walk gets longer, increase the number of repetitions you do, building to six. These bursts of speed increase your heart rate, help you work through the pain of intense anaerobic activity, and allow you to increase your speed over time. The American College of Sports Medicine also says high-intensity intervals burn more fat, so it's an added side benefit to your training if you are looking to drop some pounds.

If you live in a flat place and can't find a hill to climb, trying sprinting up stairs or stadium steps instead.

You can do cardio power exercises on a bicycle or in a pool, as well. You will benefit from getting your heart rate up and increasing your metabolism. However, to truly feel the benefits on the hiking trail, you are best off performing this routine on foot. As you get stronger, start wearing your backpack loaded down with 20 pounds. Add weight as you gain strength.

You can transform a leisurely hike into a workout by increasing your pace, adding intervals, or carrying a load in your backpack.
MOLLY ABSOLON

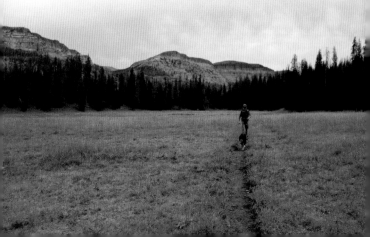

Endurance (Saturday)

Saturday is the day you want to spend a few hours training. Your very best option will be to go for a hike wearing your backpack. Again, plan to build up the number of miles you walk and the amount of weight you carry. If you are coming into this regimen off the couch, start with an hour-long walk carrying a 10-pound pack and wearing the boots or hiking

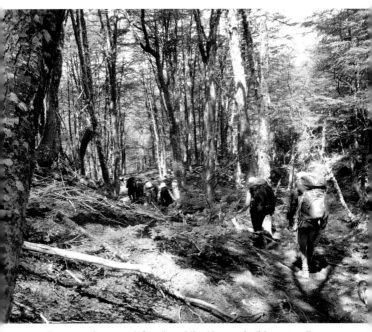

Save one day a week for a long hike. You can build up your distance, but to maximize the effectiveness of the workout, hike in the shoes you plan to wear on your trip and carry weight in your backpack. MOLLY ABSOLON

Trekking Poles

More and more people are hiking with trekking poles these days. The reason? They are a great way to reduce the impact on your joints as you hike, and they increase your overall stability. Suddenly you have the equivalent of four legs instead of two. Trekking poles allow you to get your arms, shoulders, and core into the action as you move down the trail and help support your knees. The only real downside to poles is when you find yourself in situations that require the use of your hands, such as scrambling over rocks. In that case poles can get in the way, but if you buy a lightweight pair of collapsible poles, they are easy to stash in your pack when you don't need them.

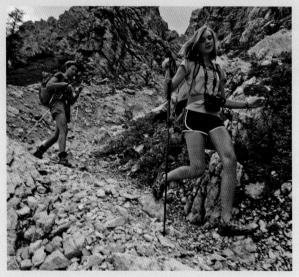

Trekking poles allow you to engage your upper body as you walk. They also provide stability on descents. SCOTT KANE shoes you plan to use on your trip. This walk should be about 2 or 3 miles long. If you can, hike over rolling terrain where you have to ascend and descend. You'll quickly find that you use different muscles for those two things. Your calves power you up the hills, and your quads lower you down them. If you live in a city and cannot get to a trail, walk the streets looking for hills.

Build up your mileage and time and choose a more ambitious hike as you get stronger. Most people are comfortable adding about 20 percent to their time each week until they reach their desired max. Your ultimate hiking or backpacking goal will determine just how far you need to go on your Saturday jaunts. You should build until you are comfortable hiking as far as you plan to travel on the most challenging day of your trip. And don't forget to think about the elevation gain and loss on that day. Hiking 6 flat miles is very different from hiking 6 miles up and down a 2,000-foot pass. In general, you can equate 1,000 feet of elevation gain to approximately 1 mile of travel. So if you are planning to cross a 2,000-foot pass on a 6-mile hike, the travel time and exertion level will feel more like 8 miles.

Cross-training (Sunday)

Sunday is your day to have fun. Pick any sport and get your heart rate up for a little while. You can bike, take a yoga or Pilates class, swim, or go for a mellow jog.

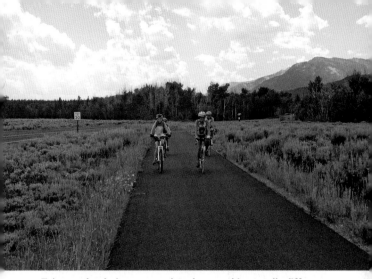

Take one day during your week to do something totally different. Cross-training keeps you fresh and brings balance to your training regimen. SUZANNE LILYGREN

Sunday is meant to be a day of active rest, so don't go all out. But cross-training is key to helping ensure you are balanced in your training and not overemphasizing one muscle group, like your quads, which tend to get a lot of attention from mountain athletes.

Rest and Recovery (Monday)

If you are training 8 to 10 hours a week, you have more than 158 hours when you are not training. This time is for rest, but in order for that rest to allow your body to recover, you need to be thoughtful about how you take care of yourself. All of your training can come to naught if you sabotage it by partying, eating badly, and not getting enough sleep.

Weight Lifting

Most of the exercises included in this book are body-weight exercises that can be done with minimal equipment. Many fitness gurus advocate integrating a weight lifting regimen into your training program as well. Weight lifting has some proven benefits. Among these are increased power, better body awareness, and an ability to recruit proper muscles to perform specific tasks safely and efficiently. You also develop muscle mass and definition, which many people desire. There are mental benefits to be gained from persevering at a tough challenge, too. Most people who feel physically strong also feel mentally strong and are better able to tackle a difficult task. But weight lifting is not critical to being well prepared and fit for a backpacking trip. It may enhance your training and in the long run is probably a good thing to include in your fitness regimen, but don't worry if you don't have access to barbells and weight plates. For hiking, weight lifting is not imperative for proper preparation.

As you establish your training routine, therefore, take time to think about what you are doing during all those hours you are not at the gym. Effective rest and recovery requires adequate sleep, hydration, and good nutrition. Try to get a minimum of 7 hours of sleep per night—more if you can. Make sure you drink enough water to ensure that your urine is clear and copious. Dark, stinky pee indicates dehydration. And try to avoid processed foods, excessive alcohol, and saturated fats. Eat a balanced diet with lots of fruits and vegetables.

If you pace yourself as you train, increasing your routine's difficulty and length slowly, you should be able to avoid feeling overly tired or sore. But listen to your body. It's easy to get excited and go at things a little too hard. If you have lasting muscle fatigue and you can barely get out of bed in the morning, you are probably overdoing it. Scale back and slow down. Overtraining can make you lethargic and unmotivated; it can also lead to injuries.

Chapter Two

Mental Toughness

Part of what helps elite athletes succeed is their mental toughness. It's the fortitude that keeps them pushing forward when they are in pain and still have miles to go before they are done. It's very likely that you will hit the wall at some point on your backpacking trip. Inevitably there will be days when you keep coming to what you believe to be the top of your climb only to see another summit off in the distance.

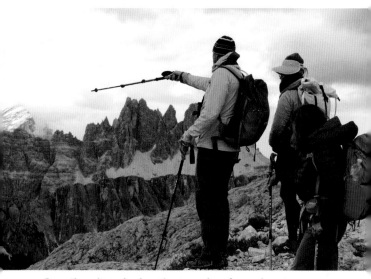

Sometimes it can be daunting to see how far you have to go, especially when the weather is poor and you are feeling tired. That's when your mental toughness comes into play. SCOTT KANE

Or you may come to a stream that is too big to cross, forcing you to hike miles out of your way to find a place where you can wade to the other side safely. Weather can also have a big effect on your comfort level. If you are wet and cold and miserable and your feet are squishing around in your boots, it's hard to push ahead with a smile on your face. That's when it's time to dig deep and get tough.

The success of your adventure is often determined by your ability to deal with adversity and uncertainty. In fact, the most memorable wilderness trips often have some hardship involved. It's when you are pushed emotionally and physically that you heighten your awareness of the world around you and feel the most alive. Many people actually seek out this kind of challenge when they go into the backcountry.

But not all of us are born with the kind of fortitude that allows us to keep going when things are hard. It hurts to push on for mile after mile when your body wants to quit. Learning to silence the voice that is telling you to stop is an important part of your training.

Developing mental toughness begins with developing confidence in your ability to succeed. You need to be able to visualize yourself accomplishing your goal, whether it is hiking to the top of a small peak or traveling 20 miles in a day with your backpack on. It's easy to undermine our potential by focusing on our weakness or the likelihood of failure. Don't be unrealistic about your abilities, but at the same time, don't

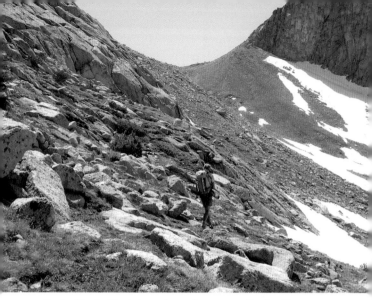

Having the fortitude to push on when you are tired and have a long way to go is what will enable you to cover more miles and see more terrain on your backpacking trip. SCOTT KANE

shortchange yourself by thinking negatively. Remember, you've done your training. You are prepared. You can do it.

The power of positive thinking is often bandied around to the point that it's easy to laugh it off as a cliché. But like all clichés, there is truth to the statement. Successful people—athletes, businesspeople, celebrities—believe in themselves. So can you. As you prepare for your camping trip, think about your strengths, focus on your accomplishments, and surround yourself with positive people to enhance your chance of success.

INTERNAL FACTORS AFFECTING
MENTAL TOUGHNESS

There are a few personality traits that explain why some people are better at mental toughness and others need to work to develop the skill. Some of it comes from your internal motivation. People who are driven to pursue an activity for their own personal reward—their dreams, passions, and desires—rather than a medal tend to be better able to push through pain and discomfort. Why? Because they want to succeed regardless of the outcome. Those of us who are looking for a prize tend to be willing to quit when we realize we've fallen short.

But you can use your fear of failure or competitive drive as a motivator. You just have to be sure you have set goals that push you but are achievable. So don't decide that you need to win your first marathon to be successful, because at mile 16, when you are being passed and that goal is long lost, you may find it all too easy to start walking. Instead, set a challenging but realistic time goal for yourself and use that to keep you moving.

The Navy SEALs have a saying: "Get comfortable being uncomfortable." That can be helpful to bear in mind as you begin to pursue your goals. You are not going to improve your fitness without pushing yourself, and pushing yourself can hurt. You are not going to complete an ambitious backpacking route

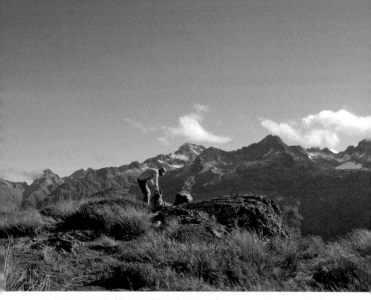

Setting a goal—like reaching the top of a pass or the summit of a peak—to determine where you'll stop and rest helps keep you motivated and moving when you start to fatigue. MOLLY ABSOLON

without a little pain, so having a plan for coping with that pain is critical. As you train, learn to recognize that discomfort is OK and can help you get stronger, faster, and tougher, but you have to find ways to deal with it. You may use time limits (a break every hour) or distance (stop when you reach the top of a pass) to help you keep going despite your longing to quit.

Finally you need to learn to control your emotions. World-class athletes actually respond to stress by showing reduced brain-wave activity, similar to the effects of meditation. Rookies tend to have heightened brain activity that comes close to panic in the face of stress. It takes practice to learn to slow down your mind when things are difficult, but the following tips will help you develop your mental toughness.

Embrace the Pain Cave

Endurance athletes learn to endure pain without emotion. It's not that they don't feel the pain—it's that they don't let it overwhelm them. They know the pain will stop when they stop, and so they don't stop until their task is over. Pain from exertion is different from the pain of an injury or illness that you don't know how to alleviate. Pain from exertion is tied to the exertion. Stopping the activity stops the pain. So you have to decide if it's worth it to keep going.

There are ways to develop some tolerance for this pain. Static-hold exercises are a great, fast trick for inducing and enduring pain. Try holding a V-sit, where you have your legs extended at a 45-degree angle above the ground and your arms extended forward on either side of your knees, balancing on your bottom. Hold this position for 1 minute. Your belly will undoubtedly start shaking and will hurt. But when you stop, the pain is gone immediately. You can also do wall sits, where you put your back to the wall and assume a seated position and hold. People can hold wall sits for a long time. Start with 1 minute and add time as you gauge just how hard it is for you. Again, your legs will shake and you'll feel like you can't hold it any longer, and then you do. This kind of exercise

Static-hold exercises challenge your mental toughness. You induce pain quickly and have to endure it without the distraction of movement when you perform wall sits and V-sits. Both exercises help you enhance your ability to tolerate pain.

AVERY ABSOLON

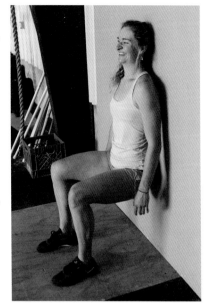

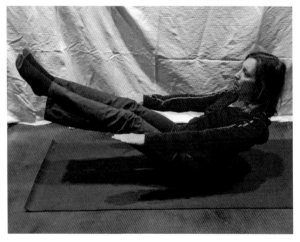

helps you realize that you can tolerate a lot more pain than you think you can.

Other pain-tolerance tricks are to do many, many repetitions of one activity. For example, in some Cross-Fit gyms the entire workout of the day may consist of 150 wall balls, where you toss a weighted ball over a line on the wall. Most gyms have women toss a 14-pound ball 8 feet, while men throw a 20-pound ball 10 feet. It takes a long time to do 150 wall ball tosses, and the repetition induces a lot of painful suffering. But suffering is exactly what you want to be doing to develop your toughness. Working through the discomfort, continuing to move at a steady pace, and persevering through the pain helps you acclimate to hard work and learn to be comfortable being uncomfortable.

Be Prepared

Part of what enables us to suffer through difficulty is the confidence that we can succeed. Sometimes that confidence comes from a coach or trainer who knows what you are capable of and is able to push you to extend those limits. Part of it comes from your own confidence in your preparation. If you know that you spent six weeks following a careful fitness program to get ready for your backpacking trip, you should feel confident in your ability to complete your goal. You've done everything you can to be ready for the experience, and you have to trust that preparation to see you through when you are having a rough day.

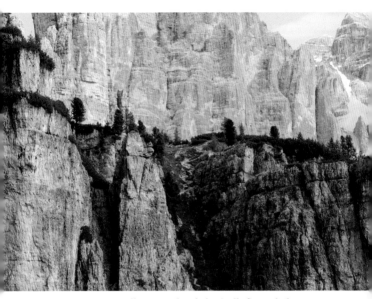

Knowing you are well prepared and physically fit can help you approach challenging terrain with confidence. SCOTT KANE

Manage Your Expectations

Having a sense of what to expect on your journey is helpful for your emotional well-being. Look at the map. Get a picture of what the day has in store for you. Are you climbing 2,000 feet over a 12,000-foot pass? Does your route take you up and down through a series of drainages where you will be climbing and descending all day long? Understanding what lies ahead and recognizing how the terrain will affect how you feel helps you when you come to that final climb at 5 p.m. after a 6-hour day. You can psych yourself

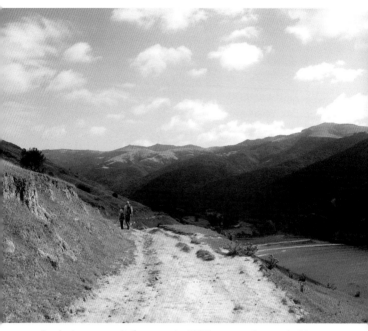

Look at your map before you start hiking so you know what to expect during the day. Surprise challenges can have a negative effect on your morale. MOLLY ABSOLON

up for one last push, knowing camp is close and dinner near. When you don't know what to expect, you tend to feel out of control as challenges are thrown your way.

Prepare for Uncertainty

While it's great to be prepared, you also need to recognize that when you are in the wilderness, you should expect the unexpected. Weather changes, trails wash out, equipment breaks, you get lost, or someone gets hurt, leaving you feeling anxious and maybe a little frightened. It's like any stressful situation that can cause your heart rate to increase and your palms to sweat. It can also compromise your ability to make well-thought-out decisions. Take a moment to calm down. The founder of the National Outdoor Leadership School, Paul Petzoldt, used to say, "Smoke a cigarette." That was in the 1960s, before the danger of tobacco was widely known, but his point was to pause, breathe, and let that initial adrenaline rush pass. Except in some very extreme situations, once the initial crisis is over, you usually have a few minutes to make a plan before you have to react. Too often when we react in the heat of the moment, we are irrational and don't make smart decisions. So slow down, pause, and think about the best way to deal with the surprise turn of events.

Chapter Three

Staying Fit on the Trail

Athletic injuries are one of the leading causes of problems for backpackers. People twist their ankles, sprain their knees, or fall and break bones. If you've put some time into training for your trip, you are less likely to encounter these problems because you will be strong and used to carrying your pack. But you still want to be careful. Getting hurt in the backcountry is a big deal. You are far from help and medical attention, and getting someone out of the wilderness who cannot walk can be time consuming and expensive, and require a lot of manpower. So be conservative.

ROUTE PLANNING

Plan your route so that you build up to maximum performance, especially if you plan to be at altitude. (See sidebar on altitude, page 58.) Remember, your pack will be heaviest and your body softest on that first day or two of your trip, so start slowly. Plan to hike only a few miles on the first day, and don't tackle a ton of elevation gain. That can come later in your trip when you've hardened and eaten a lot of the food in your pack.

Altitude Adjustments

If you plan to head to the Rocky Mountains from sea level, you can expect to be affected by the elevation. As you move higher, the air becomes less dense. There's less pressure on it, so the oxygen molecules are more dispersed, meaning you have less to breathe. For every 1,000 feet you climb above sea level, you lose 3 percent of the available oxygen. At 12,000 feet there's only two-thirds the amount of oxygen found at sea level. The effect on the body is different for everyone. All of us must go through some adjustment as we go up higher and the air pressure decreases. Twenty percent of those who ascend to 8,000 feet experience some signs of altitude illness, while 40 percent of us get sick at 10,000 feet and above. A certain number of individuals cannot go to high elevations without succumbing to altitude illness. There don't seem to be any clear predictors for who these people will be—age, sex, and fitness levels are not good indicators—so if your backpacking trip will be the first time you go up high, take it slow and do not ignore any symptoms of altitude illness.

The most obvious sign will be the fact that you feel short of breath, and exercise that would be easy for you at sea level feels difficult. You may get a headache, feel lethargic, and lose your appetite. If your body is not adjusting, your symptoms will worsen. Altitude illness is serious. If you find yourself with extreme headaches, difficulty breathing, nausea, any changes in your mental state, or ataxia (a loss of control over your muscles), you need to head down in elevation quickly. In extreme cases, altitude illness is lethal, so pay attention to your body and your colleagues. Sometimes we are better able to identify problems in our friends than in ourselves.

You can help prepare for the physical effects of performing at altitude by doing intervals in your training before your trip. Working out in an anaerobic state increases your body's ability to consume oxygen during exertion, but that will only help to a degree. Once you get to altitude, be patient. Give your body time to adjust. If you can, schedule a day when you arrive to just hang out before you start hiking. Once you do start hiking, pace yourself. Climb slowly and steadily, drink lots of water, and try to eat. Avoid sleeping more than 2,000 feet above your previous night's elevation. Give yourself time. Most people will acclimate in a couple of days.

What Is High Altitude?

High	8,000 to 13,000 feet
Very High	13,000 to 18,000 feet
Extreme Altitude	Over 18,000 feet

ON THE TRAIL

Start your day with a few of the mobility exercises we discussed in chapter one. Warming up your joints and waking up your body will help make the first mile or so on the trail feel easier.

Once you start hiking, there are a number of tricks to help you conserve energy and enhance efficiency. Try to move at a steady pace. The best backpackers are tortoises. They move slowly and evenly for hours on end, while the hares burn out early in the day. So think like a tortoise and take your time.

Plan for regular breaks to hydrate, rest, and eat. It sometimes helps to set a schedule where you hike for 1 hour and then take a 10-minute break. You can play with the numbers, but remember, you will start out fresh, feeling like you can hike forever. If you push too far during this phase of your day, you may find that later on you have no reserves and need to stop frequently. Lots of stops make travel inefficient and slow.

When you do take a long break, take off your shoes and soak your feet in a stream or lie down and elevate them. This helps to revive your feet and can give you more miles of comfortable walking.

Try using the rest step on steep ascents. To perform this technique, step forward onto your uphill leg. Straighten your leg fully, so you transfer your weight onto your bones, pause, then move the downhill leg up

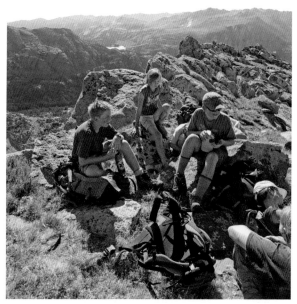

Take regular rest breaks to eat, drink, and enjoy the scenery. This will help you maintain your energy throughout the day.
MOLLY ABSOLON

and transfer your weight onto that leg, again straightening it fully to get off your muscles. This technique helps conserve energy on ascents. You can also try sidestepping as you move uphill. Sidesteps put less pressure on your calves and help spread out the work to more muscle groups. They also protect your knees. Don't forget to push down with your trekking poles if you are carrying them. That will engage your arms and allow them to help your legs with the work.

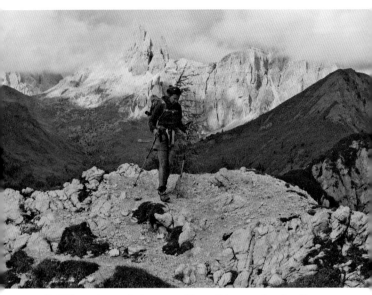

Trekking poles can help you avoid overtiring your legs by allowing you to push with your arms and shoulders. SCOTT KANE

Pay attention to your energy level as the day progresses. People tend to get hurt at the end of a long day when they are mentally and physically fatigued. So try to avoid tackling difficult terrain in the afternoon after hours on the trail if you can avoid it.

LISTEN TO YOUR BODY

Don't ignore aches and pains. We all know there is good pain and bad pain. Good pain comes from working hard. You feel fatigue, muscle soreness, and, during the activity, a burn from exertion. These sensations are normal and part of getting stronger, but they should be limited to your muscles. If you start feeling pain in your joints, pain that is sudden or sharp, or pain that shoots from one place to another, that is not so good. This bad pain could be your body telling you that something is wrong. Listen to it and stop what you are doing to assess the situation.

One of the most common sources of pain for hikers is blisters. While blisters don't have a lot to do with physical fitness (although they can be prevented if you trained in your hiking shoes), they will affect your performance. If your feet become covered with blisters, you aren't going to be able to walk comfortably, and that can change your experience dramatically. Typically a blister lets you know it is forming by creating a hot sensation in the spot that it is being rubbed. If you feel a hot spot, stop and fix it. There are lots of blister pads available on the market that stop the friction that is causing your problem. Cover the offending spot with a pad and keep hiking.

If you are experiencing a new pain in your knees, neck, or back, stop and think about the cause. It may be due to something that you can change, such as the fit of your backpack or the way you are walking. If your knees are aching on a steep downhill, use trekking poles and try to sidestep to shift the

Muscle Cramps

Sometimes a hard day can lead to muscle cramps. The jury is out on the exact cause of cramping, but most sports doctors associate it with muscle overload, electrolyte imbalances, and fatigue coupled with dehydration. (The jury is out just because there isn't a lot of definitive research into the cause.) Some people seem more prone to muscle cramps than others, so you may know that you have this proclivity before you head out on your backpacking trip.

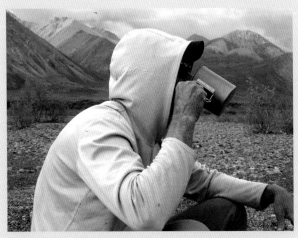

Make sure you drink throughout the day to maintain adequate hydration. Dehydration is associated with muscle cramps and can also affect how well you acclimate to altitude. MOLLY ABSOLON

In general, you can help avoid cramping by ensuring that you are fit before you begin strenuous activity. Muscle cramps seem to occur less frequently in athletes who are in good condition. It is also important to maintain adequate hydration and take rest breaks to stretch and relax your muscles throughout the day. Shoot to consume approximately a liter of water per hour of exercise. You'll know you are maintaining adequate hydration if your urine is clear, copious, and relatively odor-free. We lose a lot of moisture to sweat as our bodies strive to keep cool when exercising.

Sweat also depletes us of sodium and other electrolytes that are critical to our ability to retain fluids. Without enough sodium, we excrete water before we have time to distribute it throughout our body. So maintaining adequate hydration also requires you to maintain your electrolyte balance. This doesn't mean you have to consume a lot of expensive, sugary energy drinks. It simply means that you need to eat as well as drink when you are exercising. So try to consume salty snacks along the trail and drink water to keep your body performing at its best.

If you do get cramps, massage the muscle gently or walk or jiggle the offending muscle to help release the spasm.

pressure off your kneecap. If your Achilles tendon is starting to throb, look at your boots to make sure nothing is pressing on the tendon. Again try side-stepping to avoid overstretching the back of your heel and calf.

Anti-inflammatory drugs or pain medications can help alleviate your discomfort, but be careful: They can also mask the pain and allow you to keep moving when you really should stop if you want to avoid further injury.

Rest, ice, compression, and elevation (RICE) can help minimize the damage of an aching joint if you apply them early. If you wait too late—tough it out too long—you may give yourself an injury that takes weeks or months to heal, so stop before things get too bad.

STRETCHING

After you stop and take off your backpack at camp, take a minute to stretch. You can do simple things like circling or swinging your arms, twisting your torso, doing a gentle forward bend to touch your toes, and rolling your ankles back and forth. Maybe do a few sun salutations or other gentle yoga moves. These stretches should feel good and help you relax after a long day.

Chapter Four

Food for Health and Energy

There are tons of different diets out there. They each tend to have vocal adherents who swear by a particular eating regimen, saying it helps you lose weight, feel better, have nicer skin and hair, be stronger and sexier, you name it. Of course, these same diets go in and out of vogue quickly. This book does not advocate any specific diet, nor does it pretend to address everyone's particular dietary needs. You know your body. You know what works best for you. The goal of this book is to address the human body's needs for peak performance. You can use those principles to address your own particulars.

CARBS, FATS, AND PROTEINS

Our nutritional building blocks are made up of carbohydrates, fats, and proteins. We need a balance of all three of these components to maintain our health and energy. Nutrition experts recommend that we fill most of our calorie needs with fruits and vegetables, followed by whole grains and protein.

Carbohydrates contain four calories per gram and should make up 50 to 60 percent of our daily dietary requirements. Carbs contain the most glucose of our daily nutrients and are our body's main source of quick fuel. For athletic performance, carbs are important, but they don't have a great reputation. Most of that is due to the fact that there are a lot of bad carbohydrates out there—cakes, cookies, candies, soda, and highly processed grains found in white bread or pasta, to name a few—that give us a sudden rush of sugar but do little to help fuel us for the long haul. But complex carbs are critical. These include whole grains like quinoa or wheat berries, brown rice, lentils, beans, fruits, vegetables, whole-wheat pastas, certain energy bars, and so forth. These complex carbs are an athlete's friend. We need them to quickly fire up the engine and achieve optimal performance. But even the simple carbs come in handy when you need a quick boost of energy on the trail.

At nine calories per gram, *fats* have the most calories per gram of any of our basic foods. Fats should make up 30 percent of our daily caloric needs. Fats also get a bad reputation, but like carbs, they are critical to our physical well-being. Fats allow for normal growth and development; they provide a highly concentrated source of energy; they allow us to absorb certain vitamins and provide cushioning for our organs; and they help maintain cell membranes. Finally, fats are important for providing taste, consistency, and stability to foods.

Again, there are good and bad fats. Unsaturated fats like olive, avocado, and canola oil and nuts have been shown to be the best sources of fats. Saturated and trans fats are linked to heart disease.

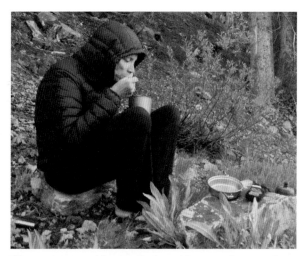

When you are exercising hard in the outdoors, you burn nearly twice as many calories as you do sitting at a desk all day.
MOLLY ABSOLON

Proteins, like carbs, pack four calories per gram and should make up 12 to 20 percent of our daily caloric intake. Proteins are critical for repairing tissues, boosting immune function, building hormones and enzymes, preserving lean muscle mass, and providing energy in the absence of carbohydrates. Protein is found in meat, dairy products, fish, legumes, nuts, and milk.

Understanding how our bodies use carbs, fats, and proteins makes it clear that all three are essential to maintaining a healthy, active lifestyle. The problems come less from consuming them than from

How much should we eat?

The amount of food we need each day is determined by our size, gender, and activity level. The range is broad, but the general guidelines say that a woman between the ages of 31 to 50 with an average height and weight should consume 1,800 calories per day if she is sedentary, 2,000 if she is moderately active, and 2,200 if she is active. A man of the same age and of average height and weight needs 2,200 calories if he is sedentary, 2,200 to 2,400 if he is moderately active, and 2,400 to 2,800 if he is active. That number goes much higher if you throw in other factors such as your environment. If you are backpacking in the wilderness where you don't have a roof over your head or a furnace to keep you warm and comfortable, and you plan to be moving most of the day, you will need almost twice as many calories as you would need at home to maintain your level of activity.

Backpackers burn between 4,000 and 6,000 calories per day when they are out hiking. That's a lot more calories than you need sitting at a desk all day. In town, you may avoid carbs and fats because you don't need a lot of energy to meet the demands of your day. Out in the wilderness it's not a good idea to short yourself on these essentials. You need the calories to perform well, feel good, and keep yourself safe.

how much and what kind we consume. The "what" kind is pretty easy to discern: Avoid processed foods with lots of saturated or trans fats. A balanced diet of unprocessed carbs, fats, and proteins—the types of food found on the outside aisles of the grocery store, as author Michael Pollan has pointed out—is the healthiest way to eat. Not only does this basic diet philosophy ensure that you consume the proper nutritional building blocks, it also ensures you get the minerals and vitamins you need.

The "how much" is, of course, dictated by several factors, but for our concerns, activity level is the most important. If you are going backpacking, most likely your activity level is going to increase from normal, so you can plan on eating more than usual during your trip. Just make sure that "more" isn't simply candy and cakes!

BEFORE YOUR TRIP

While you train for your camping trip, try to begin eating a well-rounded, balanced diet that follows the general guidelines for combining carbs, fats, and proteins. Avoid foods where you don't recognize what's included in the list of ingredients. Try to stick to fresh vegetables, fruits, meat, fish, and complex carbohydrates. Avoid sodas, candy, and other sugary foods.

Watch your weight and energy levels. If you find yourself losing weight and you weren't trying

Carbo Loading

Carbohydrates are an athlete's best friend. Your body turns carbs into glucose and stores it in your muscles as glycogen. When you exercise, you turn that glycogen into energy. We have enough glycogen stored to fuel us through 90 minutes of intense exercise, but if you plan a workout longer than that—like a full day of backpacking—you need to make sure you are consuming more carbohydrates. You've heard about athletes carbo loading; well, now's your chance to follow their lead. Carbo loading with relatively simple carbohydrates is a good strategy if you are going to be working out for hours instead of minutes. On the trail, be sure to replenish your stores by eating a snack and drinking some water every 15 or 20 minutes. And after you are done with your day, eat more complex carbs and some protein to refuel.

to, you probably need to boost your calorie intake in response to your increased activity. If you find yourself feeling weak, you may also want to eat more.

ON THE TRAIL

The principles of good nutrition are the same on the trail as they are at home. The challenge is that you have to carry everything you eat (unless you plan to fish or forage for food), and you have no refrigeration to keep things fresh.

For this reason it helps to pay attention to the nutritional guidelines you find on the packaging of your food to ensure you are getting the proper balance of carbs, fats, and proteins. In general, camping food relies less on fresh food and more on dried or dehydrated items, so you need to pay attention to its content to ensure your diet is balanced.

For short trips into the wilderness, you do not need to worry too much about the vitamins and minerals in your diet. If you are planning a prolonged wilderness trip of a month or more, it would be a good idea to have a nutritionist help you plan your menu to ensure you are not shorting yourself on critical components of a healthy diet.

MENU PLANNING

Freeze-Dried Meals

Planning your backcountry menu can be done in a number of different ways. Many people like the ease and efficiency of freeze-dried meals. If you go that route, you may not even need to bring a bowl along, as many of the meals are made to cook in the package by simply adding hot water and allowing the concoction to sit for a few minutes until it rehydrates.

There are a number of companies that make freeze-dried meals, including AlpineAire, Backpacker's

Pantry, Packit Gourmet, and Mountain House. They offer everything from chili to curried chicken to pasta primavera for dinner and things like oatmeal, granola, and scrambled eggs and bacon for breakfast. You can even have freeze-dried crème brulée or pudding for dessert. Combine this with instant coffee, hot chocolate, or tea and your cooking will be limited to boiling water every day.

There are some downsides to freeze-dried meals. Their flavor can be variable. You may want to do some taste tests before you head out to ensure you find your choices edible. You may also want to confirm the accuracy of the serving sizes. Many of the meals say they are for two, but if you are a big

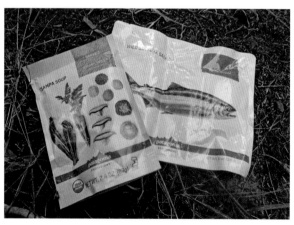

Prepackaged, freeze-dried food is fast, light, and easy. You can add protein and flavor by mixing in fish or other vacuum-sealed packaged meat. MOLLY ABSOLON

eater and are working hard, you may find the amount is a little skimpy. So check it out before you have no choice.

Finally freeze-dried meals can be expensive if that is your main source of sustenance. Prices vary from about $4 per serving to as much as $8. That can add up quickly if you are out for a week and every meal is a commercially prepared freeze-dried option.

Home Drying

If you have time and motivation, home drying food for your trip is a great way to go. You can dry everything from fruits and vegetables to sauces and meats. There is a lot of information on the Internet about drying food. In the end your results will be similar to having a freeze-dried packaged meal in that all you need to do to make dinner is add water, but the cost will be significantly reduced, and you can tailor the flavor and your serving sizes to accommodate your group.

Some people recommend packaging homemade, dehydrated meals in plastic freezer bags that you can pour hot water into, just like you do with the commercially prepared freeze-dried meals. Some people are comfortable rehydrating meals in plastic, some are not. There is no conclusive science about the health effects. The idea is to cover your meal with hot water, seal up the bag, and then insulate it in a hat or coat and let it sit for a few minutes until the contents are reconstituted. Again, it might take some

What to Look for in a Food Dehydrator

If you live in the Southwest, you can dry food using just the sun. But you need to have a minimum of three to five consecutive days with temperatures above 95 degrees Fahrenheit and low humidity for successful drying, so for most of the United States, you are better off relying on a food dehydrator.

The cheapest dehydrators do not have thermostats or timers. This is fine if you don't plan to do a lot of drying, but if you are ambitious, you'll want to invest in a dehydrator that comes with those features, as they allow you to achieve more control over conditions.

Make sure that your dehydrator has a fan; otherwise, the heat will not be dispersed evenly and you'll have varying speeds of drying. You can deal with this by moving the trays around frequently, but that can be a pain, so it's worth investing in a dryer with a fan. Ideally that fan and the dryer's heating unit should be located either on the side or the top of the dehydrator. If those features are found underneath the drying trays, they are likely to burn out quickly due to the inevitable drips coming from above.

home experimentation to determine how long things have to sit to soften up adequately.

If you are unsure about cooking in plastic bags, bring along a small pot that can serve as an eating bowl, as well, to streamline your kitchen needs. Again, it helps to wrap your pot in a coat while your food sits rehydrating to keep your meal warm until it's ready to eat, or you can let it simmer over your stove if you have sufficient fuel.

From the Grocery Store

The most popular menu-planning method is probably a meal plan made up of bulk food items. This method incorporates all different food types, and most of the ingredients are available at the grocery store. So, for example, you may have mac and cheese with tuna one night. For this meal, you can bring a foil packet of tuna, a chunk of cheese, a bag of pasta, and some spices, and you'll be all set. Meals pulled together from the grocery store shelves are probably the cheapest way to eat in the backcountry.

You can help reduce your food weight by repackaging items to get rid of garbage at home. And you can premeasure your spice needs so you don't need to bring a salt shaker or a big container of garlic powder.

Again, it helps to run through your meals at home to ensure you bring the right amount of food. If you and your partner eat only a half a pound of pasta at dinner, there's no need to carry a full pound just because that's how the pasta is packaged at the store. Rebag your food and bring only what you need. Take notes on your menu during your trip so that on

Developing Your Menu

It can be hard to plan a menu. Everyone has his or her particular likes and dislikes or special dietary needs. You can spread the challenge by having each member of your team assume responsibility for a day or two's worth of food. Or if you plan to have one person tackle the task, help him or her out by having your team fill out a survey identifying preferences. The questions to ask include:

1. Do you have any food allergies?
2. Are you on a specific diet (i.e. gluten-free, vegan, etc.)
3. Do you eat meat?
4. List your favorite backcountry meal.
5. List your favorite backcountry snacks.
6. What foods do you refuse to eat?
7. What food could you eat nonstop for the entire trip?
8. Do you enjoy cooking in the field, or would you rather just boil water?

future trips you'll know if meal X needed more spices or if you had too much rice for meal Y.

To make life as easy as possible, pack your meals for the day in a large freezer bag or a lightweight stuff sack. This makes organization easy, especially if you have to package food in a bear canister, where it can be hard to find things when they are buried in the bottom. Mark the date for each package on the outside. Then all you need to do is pull out Monday's meals on Monday, leaving the rest of your week's supply packed up.

BREAKFAST AND DINNER

Outdoor breakfasts and dinners aren't all that different from indoor breakfasts and dinners. You'll be constrained more by weight and appliances than by the actual types of food available. Most backpackers opt for one-pot meals to make things simple and fast and to minimize the weight of their packs. For breakfast this can be granola or instant oatmeal. Dinner can be pasta or savory rice. But you can bring a frying pan if you plan to be out for a while and want to add variety to your menu. Frying pans allow you to cook things like hash browns or pancakes and to bake simple breads or even pizza.

The shorter the trip, the less variety you'll crave in your menu. The longer the trip, the more weight and space become a concern, but you may also find yourself sick of instant oatmeal for breakfast every day. It's a balancing act. You can always plan a menu that includes a few more elaborate meals to keep your palate satisfied.

LUNCH

There's a saying among backpackers that lunch starts when breakfast ends and ends when dinner begins. Basically you will want to snack all day long to maintain your energy levels during periods of exertion. It's nice to have something that actually

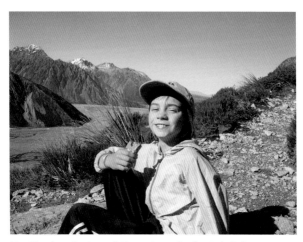

Most backpackers snack throughout the day to help keep up their energy. Energy bars, trail mix, sausage, and cheese make good trail food. MOLLY ABSOLON

resembles lunch—cheese, crackers, and summer sausage, for example—that you can supplement with snacks like cracker mix, mixed nuts or gorp, dried fruit, and energy bars.

Look for breads and crackers that aren't too bulky. Pita bread and tortillas are good because they pack easily and can withstand a little compression. Dense crackers with lots of seeds also tend to withstand packing well and provide some protein in addition to carbohydrates.

Smoked meats, jerky, and fish or chicken in foil packets are good sources of protein, although they are a little heavy, so use them sparingly. Cheese is

Energy Bars

These days, grocery stores often have an entire aisle dedicated to energy bars. The manufacturers of such bars promise all sorts of things: lots of energy, weight loss, vitamins, minerals, protein, fiber—you name it, you can find it in a bar. But is this good? There are definite pros and cons to energy bars. On the plus side, they are portable, have a long shelf life, and provide a good source of instant calories. This makes them a convenient backpacking food. On the downside, they are often expensive and can be high in sugar, sodium, and preservatives. Read the label. You want a bar that has a balance of simple and complex carbohydrates so that you don't just get a sudden sugar rush and then crash down hard when you use up those calories. Look at the calorie count. Often you'll be surprised to discover that a single bar is considered to be more than one serving, or that the number of calories contained is very high. That's fine if you are exercising and need the extra energy, but it can cause weight gain if your caloric expenditures are not matching your caloric intake.

packed with calories, protein, and fat and can be a good source of fuel, particularly when temperatures are cold and the weather is damp. Harder cheeses tend to keep better than soft cheeses, but even hard cheeses can get a little oily and soft if the

Sample Menu Plan

	Monday	Tuesday	Wednesday	Thursday	Friday	Saturday	Sunday
Breakfast	· Polenta with cheese, bacon bits, and sun-dried tomatoes · Instant coffee, tea, or hot cocoa	· Pancakes with syrup · Instant coffee, tea, or hot cocoa	· Freeze-dried hash browns with cheese · Instant coffee, tea, or hot cocoa	· Oatmeal or cream of wheat cereal, butter, brown sugar, raisins · Instant coffee, tea, or hot cocoa	· Granola and dried milk, dried blueberries · Instant coffee, tea, or hot cocoa	· Breakfast burrito, tortilla, cheese, cried refried beans, spices · Instant coffee, tea, or hot cocoa	· Polenta with cheese, bacon bits, and sun-dried tomatoes · Instant coffee, tea, or hot cocoa
Lunch	· Tuna in a foil packet, pita bread, mustard packets, gorp, dried fruit and nuts, drink mix	· Cheese, summer sausage, crackers, gorp, dried fruit and nuts, drink mix	· Instant hummus, tortillas, gorp, dried fruit and nuts, cookies, drink mix	· Salami, crackers, cheese, pretzel mix, dried fruit and nuts, chocolate	· Tortilla wraps with peanut butter and honey, pretzel mix, oranges, drink mix	· Smoked salmon, cream cheese in a foil packet, crackers, dried fruit and nuts, drink mix	· Energy bars, jerky, gorp, drink mix
Dinner	· Spaghetti with tomato sauce from a sauce mix package, Parmesan cheese	· Curried rice with raisins, almond slivers, dried vegetables, and chicken in a foil packet	· Pasta with pesto sauce from a packet, Parmesan cheese, dried mushrooms	· Rice and bean enchiladas with instant dried refried beans, instant rice, cheese, tortillas, and enchilada sauce or a spice packet	· Fish chowder with fresh fish or fish in a foil packet, instant mashed potatoes, instant milk, spices, cheese	· Fettuccini alfredo with pasta, an alfredo sauce package, dried veggies or mushrooms	· Instant Thai noodles

temperatures are hot during your hike. You can help minimize that problem by packing your cheese deep inside your backpack, where it is insulated from the heat of the sun. And even if the cheese does get a little soft, it is still fine to eat. Some people like to bring individually wrapped, single-serving chunks of cheese that you can find in the deli section of your grocery store. This approach can help you plan ahead and control serving sizes.

Sometimes it's fun to pull out a surprise on the trail when you are having a long day. Candy or chocolate can be a nice treat and can help when morale is low or you face a big obstacle and your legs are tired. But if chocolate or candy is always available, its novelty wears off quickly, so save it for special occasions when you really need a boost.

TIPS FOR LIGHTENING YOUR LOAD

Food is probably going to be the heaviest thing you will carry when you are backpacking (unless you are climbing). Your menu can add pounds and pounds to your pack weight, especially if the meals you've planned require long cooking times, lots of fuel, and extra pans for preparation. For example, in the menu plan above, a couple of the meals—hash browns and pancakes—need a frying pan and a spatula to prepare. If you are trying to go light, those items can be substituted for instant oatmeal or granola and dried milk that require only hot or cold water to prepare. For any trip, you'll want to think about your food—and the utensils you need to prepare it—carefully as you make your plans and decide if the extra weight is worth it.

One-pot meals are best for lightweight camping. Freeze-dried packaged food is the very lightest because often the meal is prepared in the package itself and requires no pot, but if you want to make up your own meals, you can minimize weights by careful measuring, packaging, and planning ahead.

Don't bring more than you need. For example, you don't need a 6-ounce bottle of soy sauce when your recipe requires 1 tablespoon. Instead, save a small packet of soy sauce next time you buy take-out sushi at the grocery store. Likewise, if you want jelly for a meal, snag a few jelly packages off the table at your favorite breakfast hangout. Little packets of Starbucks VIA instant coffee are the lightest, easiest way to enjoy a decent cup of coffee in the backcountry. These days you'll find everything from hot sauce to condensed chicken base in individual-size packets that are great for camping. You can also pick up packets for things like pesto, marinara, or alfredo sauce at the grocery store and add them to some cooked pasta for an instant meal. Dried mushrooms and veggies add flavor, some nutrients, and interest to almost any dish with barely any additional weight.

KITCHEN NEEDS

The simplest food for a backpacking trip is food that doesn't require cooking. In this case your menu would include preserved meats, cheese, energy bars, bread, crackers, nuts, dried fruit, trail mix, and other foods that don't require cooking. But for most backpackers, this kind of grazing food loses its allure rather quickly on an extended trip. There's something about a hot meal at the end of a long day that is appealing to most of us, especially if the weather is less than perfect.

So assuming you plan to cook, the lightest kitchen you can carry will include nothing more than a small pot that can double as a bowl or cup, a lightweight stove, and a spoon that can be used for eating or stirring. You can even forego the stove in some areas and cook on fires for the duration of your trip

Water Treatment

You cannot tell from simply looking at a stream or lake whether it contains contaminants that will make you sick. So to be on the safe side, especially in areas with a lot of backcountry visitors, wildlife, or livestock, it's best to treat your water. The downside of contaminated water is a pretty significant; anyone who has suffered from giardiasis knows it's better to be safe than sorry.

There are lots of water treatment options out there. The simplest is to heat your water. Contrary to popular belief, you don't have to boil water for 5 minutes to make it safe; in fact, you don't have to boil it at all. Most disease-causing organisms are killed or rendered harmless at temperatures well below the boiling point, or 212ºF. Worms and protozoa like giardia are killed at 131ºF. Bacteria dies at 140ºF. And hepatitis A is killed at 148ºF. So in order to make your water safe to drink, you simply need to heat it to the point where you see fish eyes, or small bubbles, along the sides of your pot. If you are worried about the quality of the water, bring it to a rolling boil and let it sit for a couple of minutes to ensure you've killed everything that could make you sick.

You can also use a filter, or chemicals like iodine tablets or liquid chlorine dioxide (Aquamira), to purify your water.

More recently, people have begun using ultraviolet light to cleanse their water. SteriPEN is the leading manufacturer of these handheld devices that purify water in 90 seconds or less without any added taste from chemicals. The downside to SteriPENs is that they require batteries or a charge to operate and are heavier than a little bottle of iodine tablets.

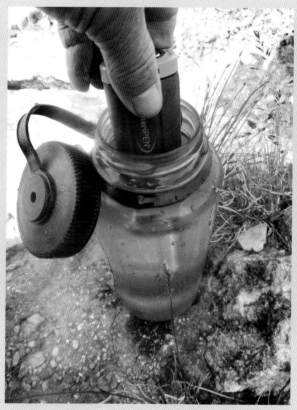

SteriPENs use ultraviolet light to purify water in roughly 90 seconds. MOLLY ABSOLON if you really want to lighten your load. Before going this route, make sure your trip is in an area that allows fires and has plenty of wood available to burn. Fires also work best if you don't anticipate camping in the rain for the duration of your expedition. Not that you can't make a fire when it's damp out, but it is certainly more time consuming than simply lighting a stove, and it can be a bummer to sit in the rain trying to light a fire when your stomach is growling.

If you want a bit more elaborate kitchen, you can carry a bigger pot that allows you to cook for more than one person at a time. You may also want to include a small frying pan and a spatula for frying or baking. These are definitely luxury items, but when you are on an extended expedition, they can provide welcome variety to your meals. Remove all plastic parts from your frying pan so you can use it in a fire or for baking without worrying about melting the handle off.

It's a good idea to bring a container for transporting water. Most national forests and parks require you to make camp at least 200 feet from water, so in order to avoid constant trips back and forth to replenish your water supply, carry something like a 3-liter MSR Dromedary bag or a plastic, collapsible water jug.

STOVES

Think about the type of cooking you intend to do as you make your decision about the type of stove to carry. If you are simply boiling water on a summer backpacking trip with a friend, a homemade alcohol stove (find directions for making your own online) is the lightest, simplest way to go. But alcohol stoves are not great if your group is larger than two, or if you

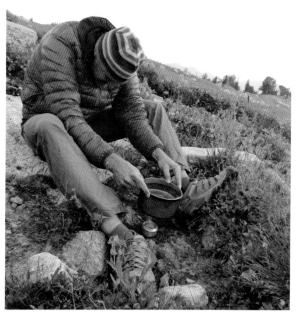

Homemade alcohol stoves built from soda cans are one of the lightest options out there for backpacking. But they really only work for boiling water for one or two people—more than that and they become too time consuming for preparing a meal.
MOLLY ABSOLON

want a little more control over the intensity of your heat source. Basically alcohol stoves have two settings: on and off.

Mixed-fuel canister stoves, on the other hand, provide an instant flame with variable intensity and are small (although the canisters themselves are rather bulky). White gas stoves are the heaviest option available, but they work well in cold temperatures (below freezing) and are easy to repair in the field. They are also the easiest to bake on if you get ambitious in your meal planning and are ideal for larger groups, for whom meals take longer to prepare.

Picking Your Stove

Things to consider when choosing a stove include:

1. Number of people in your party
   » 1–2 people—alcohol or mixed-fuel canister stove
   » 3–4 people—white gas stove or mixed-fuel canister stove
2. Type of cooking you plan to do
   » Boil water for freeze-dried food—alcohol or mixed-fuel canister stove
   » Bake—white gas stove
3. Temperatures you expect to encounter
   » Above freezing—alcohol, white gas, or mixed-fuel canister stove
   » Below freezing—white gas stove

A FEW BASIC RECIPES

Polenta with Cheese and Bacon Bits (2 servings)
    1½ cups water
    ½ cup polenta or corn grits
    ½ teaspoon salt
    ¼ cup grated cheddar cheese
    1–2 tablespoons bacon bits

Bring water to a boil. Add polenta and salt. Reduce heat to simmer. Simmer for 10 minutes, stirring frequently. Add cheese and bacon bits. Let cheese melt, stirring to mix. Remove from heat and serve.

Hash Browns with Cheese (2 servings)
    1½ cups water
    ½ to ¾ pound freeze-dried shredded potatoes
    1 tablespoon vegetable oil
    1 teaspoon salt
    ¼ pound grated cheddar cheese
    Spices/sauces: cumin, garlic powder, oregano, hot sauce,
        etc. Note: Season according to your personal preference. You'll need only ½ teaspoon or so of whatever spices/sauces you choose. Premeasure your spices at home and pack them in a small plastic bag with your potatoes.

Bring water to a boil. Place shredded potatoes in a bowl or pot. Cover potatoes with hot water and let sit until they are soft (about 5 minutes). Heat oil in frying pan. Add rehydrated potatoes and salt and fry until golden brown. (***Note:*** Do not overstir. Let the potatoes sit, checking to see if they are browning by lifting up the edge with your spatula. Too much stirring makes the potatoes mushy.) Reduce heat. Sprinkle cheese over the potatoes and cover with a lid. Let sit until the cheese is melted. Remove from heat and serve. Season according to taste.

Breakfast Burrito (2 servings)
   2 cups water
   1 cup dried refried beans
   ¼ cup instant rice
   Spices: cumin, chili powder, garlic powder, salt, etc. Season
         according to your personal preference. You'll need only
         ¼ teaspoon or so of whatever spices you choose. Pack
         them in a small plastic bag with your refried beans.
   ¼ cup grated cheddar cheese
   2 small foil packets of salsa (available at fast-food res-
         taurants; otherwise, pack 2 tablespoons in a plastic
         container)
   2 tortillas

Boil water. Place beans in a pot or bowl. Pour hot water to cover the beans; let sit until they're reconstituted. Cook instant rice according to directions on package with remaining water. Stir spices into bean mixture. Place half the bean mixture, half the rice, one-half of the cheese, and some salsa in a tortilla.

Fold into a pocket and warm in the frying pan until the cheese melts; alternatively, let the burrito sit for a couple of minutes to allow the heat of the rice and beans to melt the cheese and serve.

Note: Ideally you'll have a frying pan to warm the burritos, but this isn't absolutely necessary. You can make the bean mixture, cook the rice, and wrap them together in a cold tortilla and have a perfectly good breakfast burrito.

Chicken Curried Rice (2 servings)
>   2 tablespoons vegetable oil
>   ¼ cup slivered almonds or other nuts
>   1 cup white rice
>   1 tablespoon curry powder
>   1 chicken bouillon cube or concentrated chicken broth in foil packet (vegetable bouillon or broth works for a vegetarian version of this dish)
>   2 tablespoons dried vegetables
>   1 teaspoon garlic powder
>   1 teaspoon salt
>   2 cups water
>   1 vacuum-sealed foil packet of chicken breast meat (optional)
>   ¼ cup raisins
>   ¼ cup Major Grey's Chutney (optional)

Heat oil in frying pan. Toast nuts until brown and set aside. Add dry rice and curry powder and cook for 1

minute. Stir chicken bouillon or broth, dried vegetables, garlic powder, and salt into water, pour over
rice mixture, and bring to a boil. Cover and let simmer
until water is gone (approximately 20 minutes). Stir
in nuts, chicken meat, and raisins. Heat gently until
chicken is warm. Serve with chutney, if desired.

Fish Chowder

You don't really need a recipe for making fish chowder in the backcountry. It's so simple: You just toss in
a little of this and a little of that until you have something that tastes good. So this so-called recipe is
meant to serve as a guide that will give you the confidence to experiment. Fish chowder is a great way
to use those little 6-inch brook trout so commonly
caught in the mountains. If you aren't fishing, you can
also use store-bought salmon in a vacuum-sealed
foil packet.

> 2 or 3 small fish (any kind will do) or one vacuum-sealed foil
> packet of salmon
> ¼ cup or so powdered milk
> 1 cup or so instant mashed potatoes
> 1 tablespoon or so butter or margarine
> Salt and pepper to taste
> Garlic powder

For the most basic fish chowder, place your fish in
a pot about three-quarters full of boiling water and

cook until the meat is white and opaque. Remove pot from heat. Pull the fish out of the water and place in a bowl. Set aside pot with fish broth. Flake fish meat off bones and discard the bones. Return the meat to the pot.

In a small bowl or cup, mix about ¼ cup powdered milk with ½ cup cold water to reconstitute. (Adding powdered milk to hot water makes it a bit harder to mix in; you often end up with lumps.)

Add about 1 cup of instant mashed potatoes, the reconstituted milk, 1 tablespoon or so of butter/margarine, salt, pepper, and garlic powder to the pot of fish broth and stir until lumps are gone. Return fish to the pot. Taste. You can add more instant potatoes to make the broth thicker. You can also add other spices like thyme, paprika, cumin, etc.—really, whatever flavor you like will work. If your broth is too watery, add more ingredients.

Variations: If you have an onion, start by chopping it and sautéing it in oil until it is soft and translucent. Add the onion to the broth for more flavor. Another option is to add cheese, which will make the chowder thicker and chewier. Mild cheeses—Monterey Jack or Parmesan—are best unless you want the chowder's flavor to be dominated by the cheese.

Chicken and Sun-dried Tomato Pesto (2 servings)

10 ounces angel hair pasta (though any pasta will do)

¼ cup sun-dried tomatoes (either dry or packed in oil), cut into thin strips

1 (7-ounce) package of chicken breast chunks

1 cup prepared pesto (pesto in a tube works great in the backcountry or you can use a foil packet of dried pesto sauce available at the supermarket. Follow the directions on the packet if you choose this option.)

Pinch of crushed red pepper

Salt and pepper to taste

½ cup grated Parmesan cheese

Fill pot with water and bring it to a boil, add pasta and cook. If your sun-dried tomatoes are dry, reserve 1 cup hot pasta water in a small bowl, add tomatoes, and let sit for approximately 5 minutes to reconstitute. If the tomatoes are packed in oil, you can skip this step.

Toss cooked pasta with chicken, pesto, sun-dried tomatoes, crushed red pepper, salt, and pepper. Mix well to coat pasta. Serve garnished with grated Parmesan.

Variations: You can easily add dried vegetables to this dish to add flavor and nutrients. Asparagus, zucchini, onions, or bell peppers can all be used. You can dry your own or purchase them online. Another great option is to add dried mushrooms. Use the pasta water to reconstitute the vegetables and mushrooms as described above for the sun-dried tomatoes.

Chapter Five

Closing Thoughts

Basic fitness and nutrition are important for your general well-being, but in the context of a backpacking or hiking trip, they become more relevant for ensuring that you are comfortable and safe and that you have an enjoyable time.

Backpacking used to have a reputation for being painful. The only people who truly liked it were reputed to be gluttons for punishment. Times have changed. Gear is lighter and more comfortable, and you can find all sorts of yummy food options to keep you well fed and happy during your trip. But one thing has not changed: If you are in lousy shape before you hit the trail, chances are you'll feel lousy out there, regardless of the quality of your gear and the variety of your menu.

To really enjoy backpacking and hiking, you need to be in decent shape and you need to choose a realistic objective that is appropriate for your skill and conditioning levels. That doesn't have to be an insurmountable task. You don't need to spend every waking minute in the gym to be ready to hike 5 miles, but you do need to think about your goals and come up with a training plan to prepare you for your trip.

Backpacking and hiking are fantastic ways to experience the natural world, but only if you feel good enough to look up and around while you walk. So take the time to get ready before you go.

Index

About the Author

Molly Absolon is a former National Outdoor Leadership School instructor, an environmental educator, and an outdoors writer. She is the author of the *BACKPACKER* magazine Core Skills books *Campsite Cooking*, *Trailside Navigation*, *Trailside First Aid*, and *Outdoor Survival*. She lives in Victor, Idaho.